Home Remedies
For Blood Pressure
And Diabetes

Home Remedies
For Blood Pressure
And Diabetes

By Monica Sidoine
S.N.H.S. Dip. Herbalism

DISCLAIMER

This book is to serve as an informational guide for use in the home. The remedies and procedures contained in this book are meant to supplement and are not intended to be a substitute for professional medical care. Please seek a qualified medical practitioner for all ailments. The author nor distributors takes no responsibility for customers choosing to treat themselves. Your use of this information is at your own risk.

ISBN - 13: 978-1533545268
ISBN - 10: 153354526x

Proof Read by Jasmine Ned Anunda

Published By Create Space Publishing
United States of America

ACKNOWLEDGMENTS

I would like to thank all those who have contributed in one way or another to the completion of HOME REMEDIES FOR BLOOD PRESSURE AND DIABETES.

I thank God for giving me the vision, wisdom and good health to write this book. For all he has done and will continue to do in my life.

For the many prayer warriors who interceded on behalf of this project and also their moral support.

I thank my daughter Jasmine Ned Anunda for proof reading.

Thank you all.

Monica Sidoine.

PREFACE

The procedures in this Book was designed to be as simple as possible so that anyone will be able to follow them. Most of the items used are local things which you would either have at home, in your kitchen garden or can be easily purchased from the local market or health store for a very low cost.

TABLE OF CONTENTS

BLOOD PRESSURE

The pressure exerted by the blood against the walls of blood vessels.
Blood pressure depends on the strength of the heartbeat.
Thickness and volume of the blood.
The elasticity of the artery walls and general health.

Pressure is measured by the distance in millimeters that it will raise a column of mercury.

Systolic pressure is the highest level of pressure that exists when the heart muscle pumps blood out of the heart.

Diastolic pressure is the lowest blood pressure when the heart rests between beats.

Normal blood pressure varies from 120/80 to 140/90.

HYPERTENSION

Hypertension is unusually high blood pressure.
The blood is not circulating properly to all the tissues.
It is an increased pressure in the blood vessels over a period of time higher than 140/90.

It usually doesn't produce any symptoms until it gets really high.
Which may include headaches, shortness of breath, rapid pulse, weakness, dizziness, face turns red, pain within chest, tinnitus, irregular heartbeats, blurred vision and nosebleeds.

Common causes or contributing factors are:-
Too much salt in the diet.
Overeating, obesity.
Emotional stress.
Lack of exercise, smoking.
Intake of coffee or tea.
Heredity, genetic factors.
Excessive drinking.
Birth control pills, pain relievers.
Kidney disease and adrenal disease.

If it is untreated it can cause heart attacks, strokes and kidney damage.

NATURAL REMEDIES

- Boil a garlic bulb in 1 liter of water for 5 minutes. Drink 1 cup 3 times daily.

- Boil 1 medium chopped onion in 1¾ cups water until 1 cup of liquid remains.
  Take 1 tablespoon several times a day for several days.

- Blend 3 large celery stalks to make about 1 cup of puree. Drink daily.

- Blend one onion, 1 ½ glasses of lemon or carrot juice.
  Take half a glass by spoonful's three times daily.

- Boil 3 ½oz of sweet corn and the peel from 2 lemons in 1 quart of water until tender. Strain. Add the juice from 2 lemons and 3 teaspoons of honey just before drinking.
  The drink can be served hot or cold.

- Steep 1oz of corn hairs to 1 liter of boiling water for 30 minutes.
  Drink 4 cups daily but not at night.

- Steep 1 tablespoon dried eucalyptus leaves to 1 pint of boiling water for 10 minutes.
  Drink 8 cups daily.

- Steep 1oz of powdered ginger to 1 liter of boiling water for 20 minutes.
  Drink 1 cup 3 times daily.

- Mix 1 teaspoon each of honey and ginger juice with 2 teaspoons of cumin seed powder.
  Eat it twice daily.

- Mix 1 teaspoon each of basil juice.
  Take it on an empty stomach daily.

- Add the juice of 1 lemon to a glass of warm water.
  Drink 1 glass twice daily.

- Add the juice of 1 lemon and 2 tablespoons of dried mint leaves to a glass of warm water.
  Drink 1 glass twice daily.

- Steep 1 tablespoon of dry grated orange rind in 4 cups of boiling water for 20 minutes. Strain.
  Drink 1 cup 3 times daily before meals.

- Steep 9 soursop leaves in 1 liter of boiling water for 20 minutes.
  Drink 4 cups daily.

- Steep 10 neem leaves to 4 cups of boiling water for 30 minutes. Drink 1 cup three times daily.

- Crush dried watermelon seeds. Add 2 tablespoons to 1 cup of boiling water. Steep it for 1 hour. Strain it.
  Take 4 tablespoons throughout the day.

- Combine 1 teaspoon honey, 1 teaspoon ginger tea and 1 teaspoon cumin powder.
  Take it twice daily.

- Make a juice with 25 curry leaves and 1 cup of water. Add the juice of 1 lime to it. Strain.
  Drink it in the morning.

- Drink spinach and carrot juice twice a day.

- Drink 6oz of beet juice 3 times weekly.

- Mix ½ teaspoon each of onion juice and honey.
  Take it twice daily for one to two weeks.

- Drink coconut water daily.

- Make an onion broth with 3 large thinly sliced onions.
  Take it 3 times daily.

- Drink rice water throughout the day.
  Soak 8oz of rice in 1 liter of water for 1 hour. Strain. Add 4 tablespoons brown sugar and ½ teaspoon salt.

- Eat three cloves of garlic three times daily.

- Use cayenne and turmeric powder in your cooking.

- Eat 2 teaspoons of honey on an empty stomach each morning.

- Boil 2 teaspoons of fenugreek seeds in 1 cup of water for about 2 minutes. Strain it. Blend the seeds into a paste.
  Take it twice a day.
  It can be done for at least three months.

- Have a high fiber diet such as beans, whole grains, brown rice, fresh fruits and vegetables, oats.

- Eat 2 bananas daily.

- Eat 1 apple daily.

- Eat papaya in the morning.
  After eating it, do not consume anything for 2 hours.

- Eat guavas, an orange or a grapefruit, cantaloupe, dried apricots, raisins, grapes, and currants.

- Eat spinach, 1 celery stalk, raw onions, eggplant, zucchini, broccoli, baked sweet potatoes and winter squash.

- Take 2 tablespoons of flaxseed oil daily.

- Eat 4 ½ lbs. of apples a day for 3 – 5 consecutive days. Water may be drunk. The apples may be eaten raw, as applesauce, baked or cooked but without additional sweeteners.
  This treatment may be repeated several times a year.

- Eat the soursop fruit or make the juice and drink daily.

- Chop pumpkin leaves and sauté it with onion and garlic.
  It can be used as part of your meal.
  The stalks can also be used but due to prickles on it the outer part will have to be removed.

- Drink orange juice.

- Get 20 minutes of sunshine daily to reduce the blood pressure by 10 points.

- Rub the neck and shoulders with vinegar.

Health Tips

- If you are obese try to lose some weight and achieve your ideal weight.

- Avoid meat and animal products.

- Avoid all fried foods.

- Avoid eating junk food.

- Avoid smoking.

- Avoid alcohol and coffee.
  1-2oz of alcohol per day can raise the blood pressure.
  1 cup of coffee per day can raise the blood pressure by 5-6 points.

- Avoid excessive sweets, rich pastries and desserts.

- Check and control the level of your cholesterol.

- Decrease on the salt intake.
  Remove the salt shaker from the table.
  Read food labels carefully to check the sodium content.

- Exercise for at least 30 minutes daily.

- Drink at least 8 glasses of water daily.

HYPOTENSION

Hypotension is unusually low blood pressure.
When the pressure at which the blood travels through the arteries is lower than normal.

Some of the symptoms maybe:-
Dizziness, fainting.
Slurring of speech.
Low energy, nausea.
Difficulty breathing.
Blurred vision.
Palpitations and cold clammy skin.

Some causes can be:-
Endocrine disorders and neurological conditions.
Heavy blood loss from an injury.
Anemia, low blood sugar.
Poor diet and dehydration,
Prolonged bed rest.
Heart problems.
Pregnancy.

Certain medications such as alpha blockers, beta blockers, diuretics, antidepressants, and others can also lead to low blood pressure.

When the blood pressure is extremely low, it may cause inadequate flow of blood to organs such as the brain, kidneys and heart.

NATURAL REMEDIES

- Drink 6oz of beet juice and eat 1 serving of beets 3 times weekly.

- Steep 1 teaspoon of licorice in 1 cup of boiling water for about five minutes.
  Take it daily for a few days.

- Steep 1oz of rosemary in 1 liter of boiling water for 20 minutes.
  Drink 1 cup 3 times daily.

- Steep 1oz of powdered ginger to 1 liter of boiling water for 20 minutes. Add a pinch of cayenne to it.
  Drink 1 cup 3 times daily.

- Mix the juice of 1 lemon with a pinch of salt and sugar.

- Soak 6 almonds in water overnight. In the morning, remove the skins and grind the almonds into a smooth paste. Boil the paste in 1 cup of milk.
  Drink it every morning.

- Extract the juice of 15 basil leaves. Add 1 teaspoon of honey to it.
  Drink it daily on an empty stomach.

- Mix 2 tablespoons of honey in a glass of carrot juice.
  Drink it twice daily on an empty stomach.

- Mix 1 teaspoon of lemon juice and a pinch of salt in a glass of sugarcane juice.

- Stir ½ teaspoon of salt in a glass of water and drink it.

- Drink 8 glasses of water daily.

- Soak ½ cup of raisins in 1 cup of water overnight.
  Eat them in the morning on an empty stomach.
  You can also drink the raisin water.
  It can be done for up to 1 month.

- Consume 5 almonds, 15 black currants and 20 peanuts along with a glass of milk.

- Eat 3 cloves of raw garlic 3 times daily.

- Chew five basil leaves daily in the morning.

- Use rosemary in your cooking.

- Garlic bath for 15 minutes twice daily.
  Crush 15 garlic cloves and pour 1 ½ gallons of boiling water over it. Cover and steep for half day. Heat it and then strain. Add it to a warm bath.

- Garlic foot bath for 30 minutes daily.
  Crush 5 garlic cloves and pour ¾ gallons of boiling water over it. Cover and steep for half day. Heat it and then strain. Put the feet in the hot bath for 3 minutes and then in the cold bath for 1 minute ending with the cold bath. Repeat 7 times.

- Garlic hand and foot bath for 30 minutes daily.
  Crush 5 garlic cloves and pour ¾ gallons of boiling water over it. Cover and steep for half day. Heat it and then strain. Put the feet and hands together in the hot bath for 3 minutes and then in the cold bath for 1 minute ending with the cold bath.
  Repeat 7 times.

Health Tips

- Have eight hours of sleep nightly.

- Exercise daily.

- Avoid vigorous exercise.

- Avoid lifting heavy items.

- Consult your doctor to check if any of your prescription medications are causing the problem.

DIABETES

A disorder in which there is no control of blood sugar through inadequate insulin production. Characterized by high blood glucose level and the appearance of glucose in the urine.

There are two main types of diabetes: -
Type 1 diabetes in which the body does not produce insulin and,
Type 2 diabetes in which the body does not produce enough insulin or the insulin that is produced does not work properly.

Type 1 diabetes also known as insulin dependent diabetes typically begins in childhood. The body produces little or no insulin. It may be caused due to a viral infection or toxin.

Type 11 diabetes also known as non-insulin dependent diabetes usually develops in adults. The amount of insulin produced varies. However the individual has developed resistance to the insulin, often caused by a decrease in the number of insulin receptors on the cell.

Some risk factors are being overweight, a diet rich in sweets and refined products but poor in whole grains, hereditary, some medications.

Type 3 is gestational type, which occurs in pregnant women without any previous diagnosis of the disease.

Some signs and symptoms are weight loss, headaches, frequent urination, increased thirst, increased hunger, fatigue and weakness, blurred vision, leg cramps, urinary tract infections, gum disease, wounds which take long to heal, tingling sensation and numbness.

NATURAL REMEDIES

- Combine 1 cup of coconut milk, ½ tablespoon of cinnamon and 1/8 teaspoon of ground cloves or nutmeg. Bring it to a simmer and heat for about 5 minutes. Cool and drink.

- Boil 3 tablespoons of flaxseeds in 3 cups of water for 2 minutes. Cover and steep for ½ hour before straining. Drink 3 cups daily.

- Steep 1 tablespoon of dried eucalyptus leaves in 1 pint of boiling water for 10 minutes. Drink 8 cups throughout the day.

- Steep 1oz of sage leaves to 1 liter of boiling water for 30 minutes. Drink 4 cups daily.

- Steep 10 neem leaves in 4 cups of boiling water for 30 minutes. Drink 1 cup 4 times daily.

- Steep 6 avocado leaves in 1 liter of boiling water for 30 minutes. Drink 1 cup twice daily.

- Steep 6 fig leaves in 1 liter of boiling water for 30 minutes. Drink 1 cup 3 times daily.

- Steep 7 fresh mango leaves in ½ liter of boiling water for 30 minutes. Drink 1 cup twice daily.

- Steep 1oz of powdered cinnamon or boil 1oz of bark in 1 liter of boiling water for 30 minutes.

Drink 1 cup 4 times daily.
N.B. Do not drink if you are hypertensive.

- Boil a garlic bulb in 1 liter of water for 5 minutes.
  Drink 3 cups daily.

- Drink 1 glass of cabbage juice twice daily.

- Steep 1 tablespoon of dry grated orange rind in 4 cups of boiling water for 20 minutes. Strain.
  Drink 1 cup 3 times daily before meals.

- Steep 9 soursop leaves in 1 liter of boiling water for 20 minutes.
  Drink 4 cups daily.

- Cut off the ends of 4 okras and prick them all over with a fork. Soak them in a glass of water overnight. In the morning remove the okras and drink the water on an empty stomach.
  Do this daily for several weeks.

- Combine 2 tablespoons of aloe vera and ½ a teaspoon each of powdered turmeric and bay leaf.
  Drink it twice daily before meals.

- Combine 1 tablespoon of gooseberry juice with 1 cup of bitter gourd juice.
  Drink it daily for about 2 months.

- Extract the juice from 3 bitter gourds. Add some water to it.
  Drink it on an empty stomach every morning.
  It can be done for at least two months.

- Soak 2 tablespoons of fenugreek seeds in 2 cups of water overnight.
  Drink the water along with the seeds in the morning on an empty stomach.
  It can be done for a few months.

- Chew 10 fresh curry leaves daily in the morning.
  It can be done for up to 3 months.

- Chew 5 fig leaves daily in the morning on an empty stomach.

- Mix 2 tablespoons of powdered fenugreek in ½ cup of milk.
  Eat it daily.

- Grind dried mango leaves.
  Eat ½ teaspoon twice daily with water.

- Eat three raw garlic cloves, raw onions and string beans with each meal.

- Eat an orange or 3 grapefruits three times daily.

- Eat 3 guavas.

- Eat the soursop fruit or drink soursop juice.

- Eat greens, okras, oats, barley, whole grains, broccoli, apples, pears, cherries, apricots, blueberries, nuts, seeds.

Health Tips

- Eat a high fiber diet.

- Eat more raw foods.

- Chew the food well and eat slowly.

- Drink at least 8 glasses of water daily.

- Avoid items with caffeine.

- Avoid dairy products.

- Avoid white bread, white pasta and white rice.

- Avoid sugary foods and drinks.

- Avoid meat.

- Avoid smoking.

- Avoid alcohol consumption.

- Do deep breathing exercises daily.

- Take a 30 minute walk after every meal.

- Get 20 minutes of sunlight daily.

- Keep monitoring your blood sugar levels.

HYPOGLYCEMIA

The medical condition of having an unusually low level of sugar in the blood to a point below the minimum necessary for proper brain function.

The symptoms are:-
A craving for sugar.
Dizziness, faintness.
Hunger feeling.
Depression, nervousness.
Headaches, cold sweat,
Weakness.
Palpitations.
Blurred vision.
Sleepiness.
Lack of concentration, coma.

The causes are:-
An excess of undigested sugars, starches.
Intake of large amounts of caffeine and alcohol.
Delay in consuming food.
Smoking.

Health Tips

- Eat yam, sweet potato, carrots, mango, papaya, apples, bananas, cantaloupes, grapefruit, and lemons.

- Eat whole grains, legumes and nuts.

- Watermelon eaten with beans and avocados which will help it to not go up too high.

- Drink fruit juice.

- Drink 2 teaspoons of sugar dissolved in a glass of water.

- Avoid alcoholic beverages, soft drinks.

- Avoid caffeine, nicotine.

- Avoid meat.

- Avoid chocolate.

- Do not skip meals.

- Have meals at the regular times daily.

Other Book Titles by the Same Author

Can be viewed at this link:
http://www.amazon.com/author/monicasidoine

Home Remedies For Cancer

Home Remedies For Losing Weight

Home Remedies For Stress, Depression and Anxiety

Home Remedies For Headaches and Insomnia

Home Remedies For Sinusitis and Tonsillitis

Home Remedies For Constipation and Diarrhea

Home Remedies For Asthma and Bronchitis

Home Remedies For Dehydration and Vomiting

Home Remedies For Pneumonia and Tuberculosis

NOTES

NOTES

NOTES

NOTES